Alkaline Diet for Beginners

Top 10 Alkaline foods and herbal medicine you should be eating everyday for weight loss with plant based diet and 21 secrets to reset and understand pH right now

By Emma Johnston

© Copyright 2018 - All rights reserved.

The follow Book is reproduced below with the goal of providing information that is as accurate and reliable as possible. Regardless, purchasing this eBook can be seen as consent to the fact that both the publisher and the author of this book are in no way experts on the topics discussed within and that any recommendations or suggestions that are made herein are for entertainment purposes only. Professionals should be consulted as needed prior to undertaking any of the action endorsed herein.

This declaration is deemed fair and valid by both the American Bar Association and the Committee of Publishers Association and is legally binding throughout the United States.

Furthermore, the transmission, duplication or reproduction of any of the following work including specific information will be considered an illegal act irrespective of if it is done electronically or in print. This extends to creating a secondary or tertiary copy of the work or a recorded copy and is only allowed with express written consent from the Publisher. All additional right reserved.

The information in the following pages is broadly considered to be a truthful and accurate account of facts and as such any inattention, use or misuse of the information in question by the reader will render any resulting actions solely under their purview. There are no scenarios in which the publisher or the original author of this work can be in any fashion deemed liable for any hardship or damages that may befall them after undertaking information described herein.

Additionally, the information in the following pages is intended only for informational purposes and should thus be thought of as universal. As befitting its nature, it is presented without assurance regarding its prolonged validity or interim quality. Trademarks that are mentioned are done without written consent and can in no way be considered an endorsement from the trademark holder.

Table of content

INTRODUCTION 4

CHAPTER 1: WHAT IS PH AND HOW DOES IT AFFECT HEALTH? 8

CHAPTER 2: BASICS OF THE ALKALINE DIET 21

CHAPTER 3: STARTING YOUR DIET 29

CHAPTER 5: 21 SECRETS TO REBALANCE YOUR PH 49

CHAPTER 6: FREQUENTLY ASKED QUESTIONS 73

CONCLUSION 86

Introduction

Thank you for purchasing this book, The Alkaline Diet is the first step toward achieving your general health and weight loss goals naturally and effectively.

One of the greatest things about the Alkaline Diet is that is all based on science and what scientists and researchers have discovered about how selecting certain foods and ingredients in foods can improve health.

One of the goals in this book is to not only introduce you to this incredible and effective diet but also to help you feel comfortable that this diet can help you achieve your personal health and fitness goals, whatever they are.

The primary mechanism by which this book will prepare you for your diet is by explaining to you what the Alkaline Diet it, how it works (in terms of physiology), what you can and cannot eat on this diet, and the main lessons that you would need to know to be successful on this diet.

The Alkaline Diet is based entirely on what scientists already know about both the human body and food. Our body maintains a certain pH and foods can affect the pH of the body, causing it to be more acidic, or more basic (alkaline).

The acidity or alkalinity of the body can be detected in the urine, as blood is filtered through the kidneys to remove various wastes in the form of urine. The reason why we care about whether the body is acidic or alkaline has to do with certain medical problems, like kidney stones, than can be exacerbated or even caused by a balance shifted more in one direction than the other.

The Alkaline diet is centered on pH and the effect that pH has on the body. This will all be explained in further detail in Chapter 1.

In Chapter 2, we will delve into further detail about the Alkaline Diet specifically, namely, how the foods that we eat can cause us to develop different health conditions, as well as how educating ourselves about the acidic or alkaline nature of foods cannot only prevent or treat these conditions but improve our health in general.

In Chapter 3 we recognize that the Alkaline Diet, like any other diet, requires discipline. We discuss all of the things that you will need to do before you start your diet so that you are will prepare and confident that you will reach all of your goals. Of course, this process requires that you first delineate what your goals are before you even begin.

In Chapter 4, we will provide you with details on what you can and cannot eat the Alkaline Diet. The information in this chapter will be presented in a straightforward and easily digestible manner.

In Chapter 5, we will distill and synthesize the various details from the other chapters into 21 concrete lessons or secrets so that you don't have to do all the work of figuring out how to get to Point A to Point B on this diet. We recognize that you, like many other people, may not be familiar with the Alkaline Diet, so bombarding you with scientific and other factual details isn't going to quite be enough. What we really need to do is distill the information into secrets that you can readily digest, understand, and utilize on your new diet.

Finally, in Chapter 6 we address all of the major questions you are likely to have (and there are many when it comes to the Alkaline Diet); if you'd like, you may even jump to this frequently asked question section just to get an idea of the sort of things that most people want to know about a diet like this before they start.

We wrap it all up tight in the confusion, written to, again, synthesize the details in such a way that you feel confident in beginning your diet. We reiterate the main ideas from the other chapters, leaving you at the starting gate on the racetrack, ready to tackle your weight loss like a champ! With that, let's begin our Alkaline Diet journey with everything you ever wanted to know about pH.

Chapter 1: What is pH and how does it affect health?

Potential of Hydrogen, or pH, is one of those concepts that we are all somewhat familiar with, having learned about it in school. We have a vague idea of what it is and maybe even what it's used for.

Perhaps you know that the blood has a certain pH that the body tries to maintain, much like temperature. You might even be aware that the urine has a pH, primarily influence by all the magic are kidneys due to filtering the blood.

The question then becomes, what the heck could pH possibly have to do with a diet? Why should I care about pH at all? This question will be answered in this chapter, where we explain what pH is, why doctors and researchers care about pH, how pH can affect health, and finally, how you can manipulate pH to improve your health status.

The physiology of pH

pH is an interesting concept because even the precise meaning of the letters in this biological concept are disputed. Some say the 'p' in pH stands for 'potential', some say it stands for 'power', whatever the case may be, its importance has been acknowledged for over one hundred years, though some of the ideas underlying the concept of pH, and specifically the relationship between pH and diet and health, have been around for thousands of years. In some cuisines, including Persian cuisine, the idea that foods have a hot or cold quality, that these foods can induce certain states or qualities in the human body, and that there should be a balance between hot and cold foods, these ideas have been around for hundreds if not thousands of years. Like many other concepts, they reflect the idea that the ancients often had a very deep understanding of various states of the body and the way that various aspects of the environment, like food, can have an impact on these states.

The idea of pH, the modern idea, is the invention of two scientists working about the same time in Europe in the early 20th century. Soder Peter Laurentz Sorensen, a Danish chemist, is credited with coming up with the idea in 1909 based on his studies in electrochemistry, though he revised the idea 15 years later to accommodate for new discoveries, as, with most scientific concepts, new discoveries were always being made. Another scientist involved in early studies and classification of pH was William Mansfield Clark, who developed the early methods of measuring pH, though it is not clear how familiar Clark was with the earlier work of Soder Peter Laurentz Sodersen of the Carlsberg Institute in Denmark. In the early studies of Clark and others, interest was placed on the effect of acidity on the growth of bacteria, as many of the earliest scientists and researchers were bacteriologists. Although they were able to measure the concentration of the bacteria, they did not have a mechanism for measuring the number of hydrogen ions (the acidity or the pH) and they ended up inventing one. Electronic mechanisms were invented later on, partially as a result of fruit farmers needing aid in determining the pH of the fruit on their farms, already establishing an early link between this new scientific concept of pH and food.

So what is pH? The pH measurement is essentially a measurement of hydrogen ions, measured in moles per liter. We will not go into excruciating detail, but the pH is basically the reciprocal of the negative log of the activity of hydrogen ions. pH is dependent on temperature, with the pH of water, for example, varying significantly based on temperature. As you can see, the modern definition and equation of pH is actually based on hydrogen ion activity, not on hydrogen ion concentration, though the original pH developed by Sorensen was a measure of real concentration, which can be measured with electrodes. pH, therefore, is not an actual quantity. It is a logarithmic value. Of course, what we really care about when it comes to pH is its physiological or biological significance; in other words, acidic versus basic (or alkaline). A neutral pH is defined as lying between 6.6 and 7.3, while acidic would be 6.5 and below, and basic or alkaline would be 7.4 and up. As you probably are aware, a physiologic pH for human beings is slightly basic, which makes intuitive sense, though, of course, this is not the same for all living things as there are certain organisms that have an acidic pH.

pH quality	pH Range
Acidic	6.5 and below
Neutral	6.6 through 7.3
Basic (alkaline)	7.4 and up

[NOTE: These are ranges. In general, a pH of 7 is considered neutral, while a pH less than 7 would be considered acidic and a pH greater than 7 would be considered basic, or alkaline] Without going into too much detail in this portion of the chapter, pH varies greatly in different organic materials and even at different times or stages within a single organism. Fruits that are sour or bitter would generally have a low pH and therefore are acidic. Other fruits and vegetables are alkaline. We produce compounds in the human body that are acidic, like lactic acid produced by the muscle during strenuous activity (it is responsible for the soreness you experience during a workout). Other compounds in the body are pH dependent, like ATP (the primary energy molecule) and hemoglobin. The normal pH of the blood (human), as we already hinted at is about 7.4, therefore making human blood slightly alkaline, but again, not all areas of the body maintain the same pH, though the body does carefully regulate the pH of the varied organs of the body in order to maintain homeostasis.

The importance of pH to the human body

This, naturally, leads us to a discussion of the importance of pH in the human body, not to mention other organisms. As we've mentioned, the pH of the blood is 7.35 through 7.45, and the maintenance of this particular pH is referred to as acid-base homeostasis.

This homeostasis is very important from a medical standpoint as it can be a clue toward a possible underlying medical condition, and it also has a direct impact on bodily activities, such as respiration. Acidosis, the state of having a blood pH of below 7.35, is often caused by too much carbon dioxide in the blood, and the typical response of the respiratory system is to trigger the lungs to expel this excess carbon dioxide, leading to hyperventilation.

This is merely one example, albeit an important one, of the direct impact that pH can have on the human body and the importance to the human body of maintaining a safe pH. If acidosis is left untreated, the lungs will eventually give out, leading to no respiration at all and eventual death. Indeed, the pH of the blood is so significant in terms of respiration that the medical field has a specific test, the arterial blood gas, designed to measure it. This involves obtaining a small sample of blood from a major artery in the limbs (the radial artery) with the goal of determining accurately the pH of oxygen-rich blood from the lungs (as opposed to oxygen poor blood that is heading toward the lungs in order to be replenished with oxygen). This is why the arterial blood gas, or ABG, is measured from an artery rather from a vein. Arterial blood gas samples are quickly analyzed in order to determine the best course of action for someone with a respiratory or another organ issue as these issues are often life threatening.

Again, this is merely one example of the significance of pH in the human body. The pH of extracellular fluid or ECF (the fluid outside of the body's cells, which therefore includes the blood) as carefully regulated as part of the body's normal acid-base homeostasis.

This is not only because the organs of the human body have carefully evolved to detect and respond to abnormalities in the pH of the blood and other extracellular fluid in the body, but because various compounds in the body require a certain degree of acidity or alkalinity in order to function properly. A pH that is too low or too high may cause a protein or chemical in the blood to no longer function.

Proteins can become denatured (lose their shape) outside of normal physiologic pH and this can naturally lead to death. Many of you (the more dramatic among you) may think of the xenomorphic extraterrestrial from the *Alien* series of movies when you think of the effect of pH (specifically acid) on living things. The xenomorph alien has acid for blood and what does that acid do when it touches a surface? It burns through that surface (even metal) and would easily burn through human or other organic tissue. Now that is clearly an exaggeration of the effect that acid can have on living tissue; in reality, a pH of ECF that is only slightly below physiologic pH can be enough to denature a protein, disturb chemical processes occurring across a cell membrane, and lead to death. You do not have to be burned with an acidic compound with a pH of 2 from a xenomorphic alien in order to die because of pH. A blood or other ECF pH of the low 7's would be enough to cause death.

The Acid Ash Hypothesis

We will delve into the specifics of the Alkaline Diet in the next chapter, but the explanation of pH does inevitably lead into a discussion of how a diet can interact with pH in order to affect the human body. We have already learned that the organs of the body, including the blood, require a pH in a certain physiological range in order to function properly. We have the general idea that a pH that is too low (acidic) or too high (basic or alkaline) can lead to death (leaving aside acid attacks from the blood of extraterrestrials). But what are some specific example of, let's say, a pH that is too low?

Various societies in the United States, including the Academy of Nutrition and Dietetics, have advanced their belief that foods that are alkaline, known as "alkaline ash" foods, could be used to counteract osteoporosis, because of the finding that the human body responds to acidity by breaking down bone, increasing the risk for osteoporosis. It is believed that certain foods that are "acid ash" or that increase the acidity of the body place an individual at risk by encouraging the body to break down bone, hence eventually leading to osteoporosis. The suggestion of these societies is that alkaline foods would provide a balance.

The truth is that there is not a consensus on this issue, but various studies have suggested that acidic foods do increase the risk for osteoporosis, and these findings do jibe with the practices of various ancient people who believed that foods did have certain qualities that influence body function and that it was important for humans to eat foods that were balanced in terms of these qualities, which we mentioned earlier. Specifically, studies cite certain grains, eggs, cheese, fish, poultry, and meat as causing acidosis and therefore placing the body at risk for conditions like osteoporosis and weak bones.

The idea that specific foods are acidic and can cause the body to experience adverse effects by inducing acidosis is known as the "acid ash hypothesis" and it is the theory upon which the Alkaline Diet and some other diets are based. We will go into more detail on this theory and its various implications in the next chapter, but we will take a moment to point out that certain foods, conversely, are identified as "alkaline ash" and consuming them would reduce the impact of the "acidic ash" foods and lower the risk for conditions associated with acidosis in the body, like osteoporosis.

The term "ash" comes from early scientific work regarding the influence of pH on the health of animals. A French scientist found that changing a rabbit's diet to an acidic, carnivorous diet from a basic, herbivore diet caused the urine to become more acidic. He used a device called a bomb calorimeter to combust the foods and described that the meaty, acidic foods would leave an "acid ash" when combusted, while the alkaline, plant-based foods would leave an "alkaline ash". In other words, if one were to measure the pH of the combusted product from the meaty foods, it should have a low, acidic pH, while the basic, plant-based foods should have a higher pH when measured. Again, the idea was that eating foods that resulted in alkaline ash would reduce the risk of developing conditions like osteoporosis, and this is basically the goal of the Alkaline Diet.

Osteoporosis is not the only condition that the Alkaline Diet purports to help. The Alkaline Diet has also been suggested to have an impact on chronic pain and the metabolism of various naturally-occurring hormones in the body, like growth hormone. The Alkaline Diet has also been proposed as a mechanism to treat cancer and cardiovascular disease, increase energy, and induce weight loss. Although some have cast doubts on whether the proposed benefits of the Alkaline Diet can actually be verified, despite support from various professional organizations, the Alkaline Diet cannot be called a fad as it has actually been used medically in the past to treat certain conditions like kidney stones and urinary tract infections. Makes sense right? The kidney processes the contents of the blood in order to filter out certain compounds and actually help the body maintain a pH in the 7.35 to 7.45 range.

As a precursor to discussing some of these conditions that can be improved on the Alkaline Diet, let's take a moment to discuss the kidneys. Some of you may be intimately familiar with the kidneys while others may not. As many of you, you have two kidneys and they work in tandem to filter the blood and produce urine.

The basic operational unit of the kidney is the glomerulus, which is essentially a blood-vessel rich structure through which blood is filtered in order to remove compounds that the body wishes to remove from the blood. Naturally, a glomerulus that is functioning properly should retain those compounds that the body wishes to keep, like cells, certain compounds, and importantly, proteins. In fact, the detection of protein in the blood is one of the ways that doctors detect impaired kidney function, often caused by diabetes. In short, the kidney is essential to not only helping the body function properly but in maintaining a normal pH.

We can actually assist the kidney in its normal functions by manipulating our pH with food, and this includes avoiding foods that can cause specific problems with the kidney, such as kidney stones and urinary tract infections. In terms of preventing kidney stones (or urolithiasis), the goal is to alkalinize the urine, that is, to make it more basic, as an acidic urine (and, by extension, acidosis of the blood) increases the risk for developing kidney stones.

Alkalinizing the urine is also part of an effective treatment strategy when it comes to individuals that have already developed kidney stones. There are several ways that we can alkalinize the urine. Of course, one of the ways to alkalinize the urine would be to consume alkaline ash foods, but another way would be to avoid foods that can acidize the urine, like acid ash foods. Specifically, the phosphoric acid contained in many sodas has been found to be a risk factor for developing kidney stones (even for people that do not believe in the efficacy of the Alkaline Diet). Look at the ingredients on your can of cola. What's in there? Well, let me tell what they are. In that can of cola you have: Water, High Fructose Corn Syrup, Caramel Color, Sugar, Phosphoric Acid, Caffeine, Citric Acid, and Natural Flavor. Not only does this can of cola have the dreaded phosphoric acid (the bane of all kidney-concerned individuals), but it also has another acid: citric acid. These are two compounds that can both acidize the blood and the urine and put you at risk for developing kidney stones. Naturally, on an Alkaline Diet, you would be avoiding soda.

Getting ready for your diet

Now that you understand what pH is, why it's important, and how can we manipulate pH with food in order to prevent or treat certain chronic health conditions, it is time to talk about this important diet you are about to embark on. No diet is easy, but the Alkaline Diet is certainly manageable, and one of the takeaway points of this chapter is that with the proper knowledge (and discipline) anyone can achieve results on any diet. What's awesome about the Alkaline Diet is that it focuses on many foods that people love, foods that we may already have an inkling are better for us than others, and foods that are organic and good for the environment.

Chapter 2: Basics of the Alkaline Diet

The Alkaline Diet is a healthy and effective tool used to treat and prevent certain health conditions. The Alkaline Diet will also leave you feeling healthy and good about yourself based both on the intrinsic qualities of the foods that you are eating as well as the effect that these foods are having in normalizing your pH and helping your body return to homeostasis.

The modern Western diet is chock full of heavily processed food, starches, sugars, and other compounds that not only tend to make your body more acidotic, but place you at risk for chronic health conditions, cancer, and feeling of lethargy and reduced energy.

The Alkaline Diet is not hard to follow, as you will see in this chapter, and now that you have knowledge of pH and the impact that pH has on states of health, you are ready to learn more about the diet.

The Case of Osteoporosis

Actually, before we jump in to the basics of the Alkaline Diet, let us take a moment to examine a condition that many older Americans either are currently suffering from or at risk for osteoporosis. This is an important condition to explore further as it not only illustrates the benefits of the Alkaline Diet, but it also helps to understand how important a normal pH is in helping the body to maintain homeostasis.

Many people may not be aware of this, but your bones are in a constant state of growth and breakdown. This is not an abnormal or disordered state of affairs, but your body's recognition that it is important that the bones change and adapt, for lack of a better expression, in response to various stresses that the bones may be exposed to.
Essentially, the bones "remodel" in order to help you function as you need in your environment. The constant break down and buildup of bone can actually change the shape of your bones in response to stress. A man who rides a horse every day for years will eventually become bowlegged because his bones have essentially remodeled to accommodate the width of the horse that the rider has ridden for so long. It may seem strange, but this is the body essentially recognizing the stresses that the environment (or you as an individual) have placed on it.

This break down and buildup of bone is the result of two types of cells that are engaged in one process or another at various times and in response to various triggers. These cells are called osteoblasts and osteoclasts. The osteoblasts respond to certain hormonal triggers, which are frequently present, to encourage the deposition of the bone leading to bone growth, while the osteoblasts metabolize bone, releasing calcium and other compounds, which incidentally cause the blood to become more alkaline.

This is the reason why the Alkaline Diet has been proposed as a preventative measure for osteoporosis. As acidosis (of the blood) will stimulate osteoclasts to metabolize bone to release compounds that will raise the pH of the blood (making it less acidotic), if you were to partake of a diet that is Alkaline, you will balance out the acidosis of the blood, or prevent the blood from becoming acidotic in the first place and prevent the body from stimulating osteoclasts to metabolize more bone.

Essentially, the osteoclasts and osteoblasts engage in these cycles of bone metabolism and bone growth to reshape the bones in response to stress. This is a very clear example of homeostasis and the delicate nature of maintaining this homeostasis. All it would take to shift this homeostasis away from its natural remodeling toward significant bone breakdown is for someone to become acidotic, which can occur by partaking in a diet heavy in acid ash foods and drinks. This alone can serve to disturb the delicate homeostasis that the body has engaged in (at least in terms of bone) in order to maintain homeostasis elsewhere, in this case, the blood. As stated earlier, it is essential to life that the human body maintain a certain pH of the blood in order for compounds normally circulating in the blood to be functional and for normal processes of the blood and other extracellular fluids to continue their operation.

Acid Ash vs. Alkaline Ash Foods

In Chapter 4, we will delve more deeply into alkaline ash foods versus acid ash foods with lists of the foods that fall into the two categories, but we need to discuss this topic a little as this is the Basics of the Alkaline Diet chapter. As mentioned previously, the idea of "ash" in foods and pH has to do with combusting foods to ash and measuring the pH of the ash, which apparently was a popular thing to do in the early part of the 20th century.

Acid ash foods are those that, when you combust them, give you a pH on the acidic end of the spectrum, while alkaline foods are those that when you combust them provide you an alkaline or basic pH. The Alkaline diet is based on the idea that you can help your body achieve homeostasis as regards pH and treat or prevent medical conditions by eating certain foods. As many common medical conditions are a result of the many acidic foods that we consume in the Western diet, the Alkaline diet focuses on consuming alkaline foods as a way of treating and preventing these conditions. Proponents of the Alkaline Diet also believe that eating alkaline ash foods can improve general health and increase energy (among other things) because alkaline foods are regarded as being beneficial to the body in various ways.

It is really very simple. Success on the Alkaline diet is a function of understanding which foods are considered alkaline ash and consuming those in order to achieve your dietary goals. Naturally, you will also have to have a sense of which foods are considered acid ash in order to avoid those (and you may be surprised how ubiquitous these foods are).

Common foods that are considered alkaline ash foods include many fruits and vegetables like coconuts, pumpkins, sesame seeds, tofu, avocado, almonds, goat's milk, and herbs like mint and peppermint.

Acid ash foods are meat, fish, most citrus fruits (but not grapefruit), cheese and most dairy products, soda, and the like. Though some people may choose to consume a diet made up entirely of alkaline foods, the goal of the Alkaline Diet is actually to place the body's ECF in homeostasis, therefore the most common form of the Alkaline Diet involves obtaining 80% of your dietary needs from alkaline ash foods (listed in the next chapter) and 20% from acid ash sources.

As you might have noticed, nearly all animal products fall under the acid ash category, so a common question that people ask is whether or not the Alkaline Diet is the same as a vegetarian or herbivorous diet. Well, not exactly, though there is significant overlap and many people who engage in the Alkaline Diet either are vegetarians or become vegetarians.

There are some animal products that are considered to be part of the Alkaline diet, namely certain types of milk, like goat's milk. There is disagreement about cow's milk, as some nutritionists say that it is part of the Alkaline Diet and others say that it isn't. Certainly, if you are a vegetarian who does not eat any animal products (including milk and eggs) then you could easily avoid these products and have a full belly on the Alkaline diet since there are so many other things that you can eat.

Some people may be confused as to why certain foods would be acidic or acid ash, while other foods are basic or alkaline ash, and this is merely a function of the various components of those foods. If you think about it, when you buy food at the grocery store you can read a label to get a sense of what all is inside that food, and frankly, the case isn't really much different for foods found in the natural environment, like fruits and vegetables.

A fruit will contain various compounds, some of which are acidic and some of which are basic, or even neutral, and when you combust that fruit you may find that the overall pH is on the acidic side, rendering it an acidic ash food. The same is true for alkaline foods: they will contain many different compounds, some of which may actually be acidic, but the overall pH of the food is basic or alkaline, which is why we consider that particular food to be an alkaline ash food.

Taking pH measurements while on the Alkaline Diet

As you know by now, pH is central to the Alkaline Diet as the foods that are allowable on the diet are all dictated by the pH of the ash of those foods; also, the benefits that you hope to gain on the diet are also functions of shifting your pH in an alkaline direction.

Naturally, this begs the question of how you are going to keep track of your pH and whether you need to keep track at all, and the answer is no, you do not have to take any pH measurements.

This book will provide you will all of the information that you need to be successful on the Alkaline Diet. We do that in several ways. The first is to educate you on the ins and outs of pH, the acidity or alkalinity of foods, and the ins and outs of being on a diet. The second, and perhaps most important aspect of arming you for your diet, is to give you a list of all the foods that you can eat while on your diet.

In Chapter 4, we will list the major foods that fall under alkaline ash as well as the foods that fall into the acid ash category, so that you understand which foods will be a part of your diet and have an easy resource to consult as you embark on your diet.

Chapter 3: Starting Your Diet

This book is designed to prepare anyone for the Alkaline Diet, whether you are a beginner who has never been on a diet of any kind before or a seasoned dieter who has tried everything under the sun. Before we throw you into the specifics of the Alkaline Diet, that is, get down to the nitty gritty of what you can eat and what you cannot eat, we would like to spend a little bit of time preparing you for your diet by redirecting you inward a little. The fact is, this diet is designed to benefit you and no one else, but you. Therefore, in order to be successful on this diet, you need to have an understanding of why you are embarking on the diet in the first place.

Naturally, there may be a host of reasons or there may be only one. Perhaps you are embarking on the Alkaline Diet because you are worried about developing a medical condition like osteoporosis or kidney stones and you have heard that alkaline ash foods can help you prevent these conditions from developing. Perhaps you have heard that acidic foods just make you fell gross and you want to feel better and more energetic by trying the Alkaline Diet. There is no right or wrong reason to embark on the Alkaline Diet, but if you are going to be successful on this diet you need to understand why you are starting it in the first place.

What Makes the Alkaline Diet Different?

The reality is that there are so many diets to choose from that we would be hard-pressed even to list them all, let alone explain them. You did not have to choose the Alkaline Diet for yourself as you might have chosen from among dozens of other diets to achieve your goals, whatever they may be. In this section, we seek to explore briefly what makes the Alkaline Diet different from other diets.

We touch on this in greater detail in the *Frequently Asked Questions* section at the end of the book, but essentially what makes the Alkaline Diet different from other diets is that individuals generally are embarking on this diet for reasons that are different from those that might lead them to embark on another diet. You know why you are embarking on this particular diet, and our guess is that weight or fat loss, though it may be part of the reason, is not the only reason.

The Alkaline Diet falls into the category of a holistic or homeopathic diet, which means that it is part of a routine to achieve health benefits by tapping into a more natural life style. Individuals that are embarking on the Alkaline Diet often do have a desire to achieve weight loss, but this may be part of a general picture to be healthier, feel healthier, and to cleanse the body.

In reality, a diet is just that: it's a pattern of eating that dieters typically embark on for a specific reason. The Alkaline Diet is different from other diets as, with this diet, dieters are focused on the alkaline qualities of the foods they are eating rather than on the calories. Most diets involve various forms of caloric restriction, whether it is a general reduction in calories or a reduction of just fat or carbohydrates, for example. This is the means by which diets like a Low Fat Diet, Ketogenic Diet, or Paleo Diet work to achieve fat loss, by using caloric restriction and macronutrient ratio to trigger fat loss.

The Alkaline Diet does not work this way. Although the Alkaline Diet has been shown to cause weight loss, it does not do this by specifically targeting calories. The truth is that the Alkaline Diet often does result in less caloric intake as the foods in this regimen are generally lower in fat compared to the acidic foods in many people's diets, so this is one means that weight loss can be achieved. Again, this is not the primary means by which the Alkaline Diet works. In fact, weight loss on the Alkaline Diet is often triggered homeopathically. By helping your body achieve homeostasis more easily, and by shifting away from heavily processed foods that force the body to expend energy to digest them and which also screw around with your metabolism, the Alkaline Diet makes it easier for your body to metabolize and process foods, which can reduce fat storage and improve insulin resistance. As our body shifts to a more normal, healthier pattern of handling food (because we are eating better quality, less processed, natural foods) we tend to lose weight if we are overweight. We may also experience other unexpected effects like a fresher, healthier skin tone, improved hair texture, and the like.

This is essentially how most homeopathic regimens work. The idea is that you are replicating the manner in which your body is supposed to process foods and, in doing so, you approve the efficiency of body processes, which leads to feeling happier, healthier, and more energetic.

Engaging in a Successful Diet
There are things that we all need to do to experience a successful diet, whether it is a diet like the Alkaline Diet, or other diet types, like Paleo or Keto. Though the ins and outs of the diet may be different, in general, we all need to have a certain approach whenever we begin our journey on a diet.

The first is to have clear goals on the diet and a sense of how you are going to achieve those goals. The second is to consider consulting a physician if you have a specific health concern or you are embarking on a diet specifically to treat a health condition. The third, and this is important, is to understand what you can and cannot eat on the diet. Part of this is an acceptance that your dietary habits will have to change on your new diet. You will not be able to eat everything under the sun on your new diet, but only the foods that are acceptable under your new regimen.

This means that, as part of the preparation for your diet, you may have to make some adjustments. If you normally eat fast food for one of your meals in the day (or even all of them), you may have to begin preparing your meals, which may mean regular trips to the supermarket or your local farmer's market. On the Alkaline Diet, you probably should stay away from fast food as most fast food chains have as their staples foods that are acid ash foods, like beef, fish, processed starches, carbonated drinks, etc. So get in the habit of planning and preparing your meals. This is just one adjustment that you need to make.

Most likely, you have a kitchen stocked full of foods or cooking ingredients. Many of these foods in your kitchen may not be alkaline ash foods so you may have to consider throwing them out. The benefits of the Alkaline Diet will be so fulfilling that, though it may seem difficult to throw out or give away food that you have not been able to enjoy, you will soon find that you are glad that you did as you are now feeling healthier and better spirited than you were before.

Another general recommendation on a diet or exercise training program is to keep a log. Some of you that are already familiar with what sorts of food you should eat or not eat on a particular diet, or are good at calculating calories and the like, may not need to keep a log. For a beginner, however, it may be a good idea to keep a log or journal that lists what you are eating at various times of the day. It does not have to be anything elaborate. It is as easy as: "Breakfast: half a cup of almonds, cup of peppermint tea, half an avocado." That's it. It's literally just a record of what you have eaten. This is a good idea as it not only helps you get a sense of the sorts of foods that you are eating and how many calories you are getting in a day (if this is something you are concerned with) but is also can help you keep track of whether you are not you have actually adhered to your diet. You may find that a food that you assumed was alkaline ash, like a particular vegetable, actually is not, and a food journal will help you keep track of those sorts of slip ups.

Chapter 4: What Can I Eat on the Alkaline Diet?

In this chapter, we will discuss what you can eat on your Alkaline Diet. As we have attempted to stress to you throughout this e-book, eating healthy primarily alkaline foods is the key to success on the Alkaline Diet, and that means eating alkaline ash foods (80% of your diet) and generally avoiding acid ash foods (20% of your dietary total).

Think of acid ash foods as your kryptonite. Just as kryptonite was enough to weaken Superman to the point that he was not able to defeat his enemies, acid ash foods can disturb your body enough to trigger or exacerbate underlying health problems, make you feel less energetic, and possibly even put you at risk for serious health problems down the line and cause faster aging.

Not to speak on your behalf, but you do not want that. You want to be Superman, you want to be Captain America, you want to be Aquaman. You want to be youthful and strong, healthy enough to meet any task that you have to undertake head on.

Many of you may be familiar with the concept of so-called superfoods. For those of you that are not familiar, superfoods are healthy, natural foods that contain antioxidants and other chemicals that can help you fight and prevent illness. Studies have suggested that they can actually live longer.

Any search on the internet will reveal what some of these superfoods are: things like mango, coconut, kale, chia, avocado, salmon, garlic, the list goes on. Although many of you will not be familiar with the alkaline ash foods yet, those of you that are will notice that the list of these common superfoods does include some alkaline ash foods, namely, coconut, avocado, garlic. While there are some on there that we would definitely consider acid ash, like salmon.

The point here is that, though we may think of alkaline ash foods as "superfoods" as most of them have been shown to confer some helpful benefits that can help us to live longer, they are not exactly the same as the superfoods that you may have read on the internet.

You will have to be careful here. You want to consume foods that fall into the alkaline ash category, not just foods that are described as "superfoods." With that out of the way, let's jump right into the list of alkaline ash foods.

Alkaline Ash Food Chart

FRUITS	VEGETABLES	GRAINS AND BEANS
Oranges	Carrots	Quinoa
Bananas	Corn	Wild Rice
Cherries	Mushrooms	Millet
Pineapples	Cabbage	Amaranth
Peaches	Peas	Soybeans
Avocados	Potato skins (skin only)	Green Beans
Dates	Olives	Gluten/Yeast
Figs	Sweet Potato	
Melons	Zucchini	
Grapes	Lettuce	
Papaya	Celery	
Kiwi	Beets	
Berries	Squash	
Apples	Okra	
Pears	Garlic	
Raisins	Broccoli	
Mangoes	Spinach	
Grapefruits	Parsley	
Lemons	Onions	
Limes	Asparagus	
Watermelon	Pumpkins	
Pomegranates	Radishes	
Tomatoes	Cauliflower	
	Kale	

	Kelp Wakame Collards Chive Onions Endive Chard Brussels sprouts	
OILS Avocado Oil Coconut Oil Olive Oil Flax Seed Oil Canola Oil	**NUTS AND SEEDS** Almonds Chestnuts Coconuts Sunflower Seeds Sesame Seeds Pumpkin Seeds Flax seeds	**GRASSES** Oat Grass Shave Grass Dog Grass Kamut Grass Barley Grass Wheatgrass
DAIRY Soy Milk Goat Milk Whey Breast Milk	**SWEETENERS** Raw Honey Raw Sugar Maple Syrup Rice Syrup	**OTHER** Tofu Ginger Tea Green Tea Herbal Teas

	Stevia	Mint
		Peppermint
		Buckwheat pasta
		Alkaline Water
		Sauerkraut

Those were your alkaline ash foods and, as you can see, there are a lot of them so don't worry, this diet isn't like being thrown into a prison in a faraway country. You can easily formulate a meal plan for the day that will easily allow you to prepare all of your meals at home from ingredients purchased from your local grocery store or farmer's market. You can even eat out if that is important to you. You will have plenty to choose from! Up next on the roster (of the opposing team), we have the acid ash foods. These are the foods that you should limit while on the Alkaline Diet.

Acid Ash Food Chart

FRUITS	VEGETABLES	GRAINS AND BEANS
Prunes	Cooked Spinach	
Cranberries	Potatoes (without the skin)	Brown Rice
Blueberries		Spelt
Rhubarb		Sprouted Wheat
Sour Cherries		Rye
Processed Fruit		Oats
Juices		Buckwheat
Plums		Cooked Corn
		White Rice
		Pasta
		Pastries
		White Flour
		Wheat
		Barley
		String Beans
		Kidney Beans
		Lima Beans
		Navy Beans
		Pinto Beans
OILS	**NUTS AND SEEDS**	**GRASSES**

Corn Oil	Sunflower Seeds Pumpkin Seeds Cashews Pecans Walnuts Peanuts	Wheat Germ
DAIRY Cottage Cheese Buttermilk Yogurt Butter Eggs Raw Milk Ice Cream Homogenized Milk Cheese	**MEATS** Fish Venison Lamb Chicken Turkey Shellfish Pork Beef	**OTHER** Non-herbal teas (and teas not listed in the alkaline ash chart) Coffee Soft Drinks and Sodas Beer Chocolate Molasses Processed Honey Brown Sugar White Sugar Sweet N' Low Aspartame Equal

		NutraSweet
		Wheat Germ
		Soda Crackers

A standard version of the Alkaline Ash Diet states that we should consume 80% alkaline ash foods and 20% acid ash foods, so plan accordingly. Again, some people may choose to consume a diet that is entirely alkaline.

Top 10 Alkaline Foods You Should Be Eating Everyday

1 – Spinach

Spinach Spinach is a powerful vegetable that has many health characteristics, including its alkaline effects. This is largely due to it's high content of chlorophyll, which causes the spinach to be an alkalizing agent to the body and restore the pH level back to its ideal. Along with its alkalizing properties, spinach is loaded with essential vitamins and minerals, including: Vitamin A, Vitamin C, Vitamin K, Vitamin E, Vitamin B2, Magnesium, Iron, Calcium, Folate, Manganese and Potassium. Because of this, spinach alone can help the body to feel better and run at a better capacity. It prevents anemia, heart disease, signs of aging, cancer, muscle weakness and skin damage. For best results, be sure to consume at least one cup of spinach daily, either raw, cooked or blended into a smoothie.

2 – Lemons

This may be surprising, as lemons are often seen as an acidic fruit. However, they are actually high in alkaline properties. This is because once the citric acid in lemons are metabolized, they provide an alkaline effect on the body. They help to cleanse and detox the body, using essential minerals like calcium and iron. Lemons aid the body in proper functioning of the digestive system and immune system. They also help one to lose weight, control their blood pressure and fight off cancerous cells. In order to fully benefit from lemons, be sure to consume a lemon water mixture first thing in the morning, on an empty stomach. Simply mix the juice from one half of a lemon with a glass of lukewarm water. Then, wait at least thirty minutes prior to consuming food.

3 – Kale

Kale is another powerful green that should be added to a daily diet. It has the ability to stabilize the body's pH levels, while providing detoxification and antioxidant properties. Kale contains Vitamin A, Vitamin K, Vitamin C, Magnesium, Calcium, Copper, Potassium, Iron, Protein, Phosphorus and Manganese. With all of these healthy characteristics, it is no surprise that research has shown that kale can help to reduce cholesterol, to reduce blood pressure, to lose weight and to reduce the risk of cancer. Be sure to consume approximately two cups of kale at least four times per week to fully reap its benefits.

4 – Avocados

Avocados are another one of those foods that are packed with essential vitamins and minerals that help to flush out harmful toxins from the body and help to restore the body's pH level to its optimum level. By doing so, avocados help the cardiovascular system, the immune system, the circulatory system and the digestive system. Since avocados are so beneficial to the body, it is recommended to consume them on a daily basis. Try to consume at least half an avocado each day. They are delicious and can be added to almost any dish or smoothie.

5 – Wheatgrass

Wheatgrass also helps to detoxify the body. In doing so, it also helps to protect the liver from harmful toxins. Since it contains essential vitamins and minerals, along with ridding the body of toxins that weigh it down, wheatgrass helps to boost energy, lose weight, stabilize blood sugar and fight cancerous cells. Wheatgrass can be consumed in several forms: juiced from the raw plant or bought in powder form. If juiced, consume one to two ounces daily. If using powder form, add one teaspoon to a glass of water and consume each day.

6 – Celery

Celery is a healthful food that is not given the credit it is deserved. Celery is normally found on every diet's menu. This is largely because celery is a diuretic, as it helps the body to get rid of any excess fluids. Celery can also neutralize the acid in the body and bring the pH level back to a slightly alkaline level. Celery alone can keep the body in an alkaline state. So, consume 2 to 3 stalks of celery per day and the pH level should sit comfortably at the ideal 7.40.

7- Broccoli

Broccoli is one of the most important foods to eat in order to maintain an alkalized pH levels. That is because broccoli contains phytochemicals that alkalize the body, reduce estrogen dominance and increase estrogen metabolism. Broccoli also contains antioxidants and anti-inflammatory properties. It is able to improve the digestive system, the cardiovascular system, the immune system and the integumentary system. This is largely because of the vitamins and minerals that broccoli contains, which includes: Vitamin A, Vitamin K, Vitamin C, Iron, Folate, Protein, Fiber,

Manganese, and Potassium. To fully benefit from broccoli's healthy properties, be sure to consume it at least four times per week. Try it either steamed or roasted, for best results.

8 – Cucumbers

Cucumbers are another food that have a high water content and help to flush out harmful toxins from the body. They can help to restore the pH level of the body by neutralizing the acids. They also help to reduce any inflammation within the body. Cucumbers are a fantastic source of vitamins and minerals and therefore should be consumed on a regular basis. They are low in calories and help to keep the body hydrated. They are an excellent addition to any healthy eating plan. Cucumbers help to improve heart health, blood sugar levels, digestion and ridding the body of excess weight. They can even help fight cancerous cells.

9 – Bell Peppers

One highly underestimated food is the bell pepper. Not only can the bell pepper help to neutralize the acid in the body and raise the pH level to alkaline, but it can help to reduce anxiety, lower blood pressure, reduce inflammation, and fight cancer. Consume at least one cup of bell peppers three to four times per week. They can be eaten raw, roasted, grilled or baked.

10 – Garlic

Like many contained in this list, garlic has so many healthy characteristics that go far beyond restoring the pH level in the body. Garlic helps to support the body's overall health. It contains Vitamin B1, Vitamin B6, Vitamin C, Calcium, Copper, Selenium and Manganese. It acts as an antibacterial food, an antiviral food, an antioxidant food, and an anti-fungal food. In order to experience the benefit of neutralizing the body's acids and restoring the pH level, the garlic must be crushed or chopped. This is because it is essential to release important sulfur compounds. Eat two to four fresh garlic cloves each day and the body's pH level will stabilize.

Chapter 5: 21 Secrets to Rebalance Your pH

Now that you have an understanding of the basic of the Alkaline Diet and also have an idea of what foods are the mainstay of your diet, you are ready to tackle your diet head-on. You will do that by learning the 21 secrets that are the keys to success on the Alkaline Diet.

These secrets will not only aid you in better understanding the diet but reiterate the main concepts that are essential to entering your diet like Clark Kent and leaving it like Superman. It really isn't that difficult.

Secret 1: Understanding what pH is and how it works is the key to creating a normal balance in the human body and encouraging overall health. The human body seeks to maintain a certain homeostasis and specific foods that we eat can either encourage the body's natural homeostasis or derail it.

The key to achieving success on the Alkaline Diet is having an understanding of what pH is and why it is important to your health.

Sure, most of us would have learned about pH in school, but that was a long time ago for many of you and one of the goals of this book is to take what you know (and maybe what you don't) and help you to redirect that information towards a healthy, happier lifestyle.

Though you do not need to measure pH of urine or other bodily fluids to achieve success on this diet, you do need to have a basic understanding of what's in foods and why it's important. Fortunately for you, we have done most of that work for you by distilling all of that information into the two charts that you read in the previous chapter.

Secret 2: The normal pH of the human body lies between 7.35 and 7.45. A blood pH below 7.35 is described as acidotic while a blood pH above 7.45 is described as alkaline or basic.

This is not a science book and you do not have to memorize any calculations in order to be successful on the Alkaline Diet.

What is it important to know, however, is that there is something called physiologic pH, and that is the natural pH that the body seeks to maintain in the blood and other extracellular fluids in order for it to engage in its normal bodily processes and achieve homeostasis.
The pH will vary depending on the type of extracellular fluid, but the normal pH for the blood is about 7.4.

Remember, the body needs to maintain this pH in order for proteins and other compounds in the blood to maintain their normal shape; this pH is also important for cells in the blood and lining the blood to engage in their normal metabolic and other processes.
The body actually has to expend energy to maintain this pH as this pH is necessary for life to continue.

Secret 3: Even the ancients understood the importance of consuming foods that contained a certain
balance between the specific qualities of the food. The Alkaline Diet is based on the same idea.

Although the Alkaline Diet of today is based on science that was not well understood until the beginning of the early 20th century, the underlying concepts of this diet date back thousands of years. Even the ancients under the ideas of "humors" or physical qualities of the blood and body that could either cause illness or prevent it.

Essentially, scientists and thinkers of the past were talking about pH and other chemical qualities of the blood and body that we did not begin to understand until the 20th century. These ancient minds were able to treat illnesses that even today we have difficulty fully treating or even understanding with solely well-thought out diet regimens.

They were perceptive in ways that we can hardly imagine, and people in the past were able to live long, healthy lives on natural alkaline food sources like olive oil, fruits, vegetables, grains, and grasses.

Secret 4: The Alkaline Diet of today is based on the magical ratio of 80% alkaline ash foods and 20% acidic foods. The Alkaline Diet of today, that we advocate for in this book, consists of partaking of a diet that is made up of 80% alkaline ash foods and 20% acid ash foods.

Though some people choose to partake of a diet that is made up exclusively of alkaline ash foods, this is not necessary on this diet. Therefore, you will be able to partake of *some* meat, fish, or eggs (and other acidic spectrum foods) if you really want to! What's great about the alkaline ash diet, and contrary to what some people might think, is that there are many delicious, exciting foods that you can partake of in this diet. It's not your grandmother's cod liver oil and prunes (both of which are acidic, by the way), this is a diet that you can easily convert into delicious meals every day.

This is especially easy in this day and age where foods and food products from around the world are more readily available than they have ever been before. Before we dive into the next secret on the list, let's spend a moment to talk about some of these delicious foods. We have made a list of ten foods that you can incorporate into almost any meal to maintain the alkalinity of that meal.

Wheatgrass. It is simple and easy to incorporate a shot of wheatgrass into any meal, or even to have a shot at different times of the day. Wheatgrass is easily obtained at grocery stores and health food stores and it only takes a few shots here and there to obtain the varied health benefits associated with this awesome, easy alkaline food.

Tofu. Tofu is not only healthy and affordable, it can be used as an ingredient in a wide variety of foods. Made from soybeans, tofu is more readily available than ever before. You can fry eat, eat it plain, use it to make tofu burgers. The possibilities really are endless with tofu, a miracle food and a staple of the Alkaline Diet for many people.

Almonds. The great thing about almonds and nuts is that they are a dry food that it is easy to transport and snack on. And you don't have to snack on them, they can be an intrinsic part of a meal, like a salad, a vegetable dish, the list goes on. Not only that, almond milk is also derived from almonds and almond milk is a favorite for people who are either lactose intolerant or wish to keep things alkaline by staying away from animal milks (though goat's milk is considered an alkaline ash food). Many recipes these days incorporate almond milk so if you are really committed to this diet, almonds and almond milk are an ingredient that you should make great use of.

Grapefruit. Grapefruit is not only delicious, but it is easily obtainable and healthy. There was a time when people loved to snake on fruits like grapefruit, and though it may seem like those days are far in the past they do not have to be. Incorporating grapefruit into your 80% alkaline ash foods for the day will help you to easily meet your daily requirements.

Sesame Seeds. Sesame seeds are an easy alkaline ash food that can be incorporated into any food. They taste great, their easy to obtain, and their cheap. Consider having sesame seeds in your kitchen as part of your new Alkaline Diet regimen.

Tomatoes. Tomatoes are an alkaline food that many of you probably already manage to incorporate into your meals. They can easily be added to a salad or tofu burger; they can even be eaten as a snack.

Coconut. Coconuts are widely considered to be a superfood, not only because they are so healthy, they are also delicious and can be utilized in a variety of different ways, allowing them to be incorporated into many meals and recipes.

Coconuts can certainly be eaten in their natural form, but they can also be consumed in the form of coconut juice, coconut oil, coconut milk and the like. Coconuts are truly a miracle food and we recommend the coconut as a staple of your Alkaline Diet.

Avocados. Avocados are another so-called superfood and these should also be incorporated into your Alkaline Diet. They can be incorporated into many dishes and meals or they can be eaten alone. When you embark on the Alkaline Diet, you begin to realize how fulfilling it is to engage in a diet that's just as delicious and filling as a modern diet, but without all the chips and soda. You can go to sleep at night knowing that you ate heartily and well. And all it took was an avocado...

Pumpkins. Sure there are lots of things that you can do with a pumpkin, and one of the best is eating one. It does not have to be Halloween for you to enjoy the company of a pumpkin. Put some on your salad or include it with a great vegetable dish. Incorporate a pumpkin into your life today.

Watercress. All right, watercress sprouts are one of those things that you always hear about, but never manage to incorporate into your diet, but you should. They can easily be incorporated into a variety of meals. They are also low in calories and confer some great nutritional benefits. Make friends with the watercress today!

Secret 5: An Alkaline Diet can be used to treat conditions associated with acidosis of the blood or urine, including kidney stones, urinary tract infections, and osteoporosis.

This is a poorly-kept secret. Many of you embarking on the Alkaline Diet are doing so because you may be knee deep in a particular health problem and you have heard that the Alkaline Diet can help you remedy that problem.

As we have reiterated many times in various locations in this book, many health problems are directly related to consuming diets that are heavy in acid ash foods. Not only that, but many detrimental states in the body cause the blood to become shifted towards acidosis, causing the body to have to work overtime to maintain a homeostasis that is not only natural, but essential for life.

In reality, you do not have to be suffering from any ailment to derive benefit from the Alkaline Diet. Many people choose to partake of this diet because they want to prevent illness or medical conditions that develop later in life like osteoporosis.

Secret 6: The human body goes to great lengths to maintain homeostasis, as certain conditions (which we can summarize as homeostasis) are essential for the body to function normally.

This is another concept that is important to reiterate because it is not only an important part of the Alkaline Diet, but it is also a secret that even people in the medical community do not understand.

Though the Alkaline Diet may be unique compared to other diets, it also shares some commonalities with them. Many modern diets of day work by understanding how the body works normally. For example, the Intermittent Fasting diet works by tapping into how the human body normally processes food after centuries of evolution. The human body has evolved to expect periods of fasting (when one is not eating) punctuated by periods of eating. When you are not eating, the body burns fat from its own fat stores to meet its caloric requirement. This is an example of how a diet can tap into how the body functions normally. Well, the Alkaline Diet isn't much different.

The Alkaline Diet taps into your body's own desire to maintain homeostasis by helping your body get there. Because you are assisting your body in this process, your body does not have to deal with the confusion of all of these acid ash foods flooding the bloodstream when you are already acidotic to begin with; now your body not only has to digest these heavily-processed acid ash foods, but it also has to try to shift your bloodstream towards alkalinity, and god forbid you have a kidney stone…

Essentially, consuming a diet heavy in acid ash foods is a mess for the body, especially if you are an older individual, overweight, or already have health problems. Homeostasis is a state that your body goes to great length to reach and you can be a bro and help your body along a little bit.

Secret 7: A simple way of conceptualizing the Alkaline Diet is to think of it as a means that you can help your body achieve homeostasis by avoiding the typically acid ash foods of the Western diet and partaking in foods that shift the body away from acidosis.

The goal of this "secret" is merely to help you understand why the Alkaline Diet is more than a diet; it's a way of life. This diet is not merely a means for you to lose weight or achieve this goal or that. The Alkaline Diet is a way to help your body function normally, reduce your risk for various health problems down the line, increase your energy, and possibly even increase longevity.

Secret 8: The Alkaline Diet can be used to prevent osteoporosis in older individuals by reducing the acidosis of the blood thereby discouraging the body from metabolizing bone and *encouraging bone deposition.*

Good old Osteoporosis. Our old friend. The reason why we keep bringing it up is because this condition really represents one of the best examples of how the Alkaline Diet can change people's lives. It is also an example that illustrates that the Alkaline Diet isn't just another hokey diet, like some other diets that we will not name here.

The Alkaline Diet is grounded in understanding the importance of pH in maintaining health and preventing the development of health conditions down the line. Though many people around the world will develop osteoporosis through no fault of their own, there are things you can do to help with your osteoporosis diagnosis or to at least delay it if you are getting close an age to this dreaded condition.

One of the ways that your body helps to maintain a homeostatic pH is by mobilizing alkaline substances from various parts of the body to raise the pH, and one of those locations is the bone. If you are already helping your body to be more alkaline, then you reduce the risk of your body mobilizing bone to fix the pH of the blood, and you also encourage the body to deposit bone rather than break down. This is a secret of the Alkaline Diet. This diet can actually push your body towards bone deposition rather than bone breakdown.

Secret 9: The Alkaline Diet can trigger weight loss as "alkaline ash" foods are often lower in calories than acid ash foods and frequently contain healthy antioxidants.

Although the primary goal of a dieter on the Alkaline Diet often is not weight loss, you can help push your body towards weight loss merely by consuming foods that are in the proper ratio of 80% from alkaline ash sources and 20% from acid ash sources.

Again, what's great about this diet is that it comes with a host of unexpected advantages that most dieters were not thinking about when they decided on to embark on this diet. You may have set sail on the Alkaline Diet thinking that you would prevent yourself from developing those painful kidney stones that you know run in the family, and, inadvertently, your skin has improved, your hair is thicker and shinier, you've lost some of that stubborn belly fat, and you might even have lengthened your life span. These are all things that you would have to be a fool to say "No" to.

Secret 10: Before you begin any diet, it is important to make a list of everything you hope to achieve while on your diet. This will both motivate you to continue your diet when times get a little rough, while also helping you to measure whether or not you are achieving the success you hoped for on your diet.

This is a secret that applies to any diet, but it is particularly important on this one as, for many of you, at least, your goal may not be purely weight loss.

The good thing about having weight loss as a goal is that it should be relatively easy to tell if you are meeting this goal or not, right? You weight yourself one week in, two weeks in, three weeks in, etc. and you should be able to quantify if you are losing weight or not. As many people on this diet will have other reasons for why they chose this one over others it will be important for you to keep track of whether or not you are meeting these goals. This is not only for practical reasons: what's the point of going to the farmer's market twice a week to get pomegranates and wheatgrass if you have no idea that the diet is working because you don't remember why you decided to go on it on the first place?

Don't get me wrong. It is perfectly all right to embark on a diet merely because you want to live a healthy lifestyle. Frankly, that is one of the better reasons to go on a diet. But if you did have specific reasons as to why you chose this diet, it would be important to keep track of those somehow, wouldn't it? That's a key secret to success on any diet.

Secret 11: The Alkaline Diet is good for the environment. If you take a hop and a skip back to the last chapter, you will see that the Alkaline Diet is very heavy in natural ingredients that come from natural sources.

Recall that the Alkaline Diet does not involve any products that come from meat or fish flesh, and the only dairy products are certain types of milk (and the occasional cheese). As many of the world's current environmental problems stem from the industrialization of farming with huge farm operations where cows and chickens and other animals are pumped full of hormones which is why that drumstick you got at KFC looked like it was sponsored by Arnold Schwarzenegger or Dwayne Johnson or something because it was so insanely jacked.

You are avoiding these industrialized type of foods in favor of things that you can get at a farmer's market or the produce section of your grocery store. Therefore, by embarking on the Alkaline Diet you are not only doing good for yourself, but for this planet that we all must share.

Secret 12: Although the Alkaline Diet may be different from other diets because the goal is not necessarily weight loss, it still requires discipline as the modern American diet contains many foods that are considered acid ash foods.

The secret to success on this diet is discipline. Many diets fail because the dieter is not disciplined in enough to stick to it. Oftentimes, this is a function of the diet itself. Perhaps the diet is too difficult to embark on, or perhaps the instructions or requirements of the diet are too complicated to follow easily.

In this book, we have attempted to avoid this particular dietary pitfall by providing you with everything that you need to be successful on this diet. We have provided you with the information needed to understand the diet, we have given you a list of alkaline ash and acid ash foods. But, at the end of the day, we cannot consume this diet for you. It is still your diet for you to be successful on, and that success will require some discipline on your part.

Secret 13: Most diets that dieters engage in utilize total caloric restriction in order to achieve weight loss. In other words, dieters typically have to restrict their calories in order to achieve the weight loss they desire. Although the Alkaline Diet often does result in lower caloric intake, the mainstay of this diet is not an intentional restriction of calories, but a focus on foods that alkalinize the blood and urine.

What's great about this diet is that dieters can achieve their goals without deliberately restricting their calories. Though your primary goal may be weight loss (and it's okay if it isn't), you will find that you will achieve both total weight loss and fat loss on the Alkaline Diet. When your body begins to behave in a more efficient manner, a typical result is that you tend to shift toward your natural body weight, which for many people in the Western World is a lower weight than where they are currently.

Therefore, merely by following an Alkaline Diet closely (as you should) you will find that you will not only achieve those goals that you listed when you began this diet, but that you will also start to see the pounds fall off.

Secret 14: Make a list of the foods that you can eat on this diet.

All right, so we did the hart part, which is to make a list of all the alkaline ash foods from which you should draw in order to get 80% of your daily calories on this diet, but we cannot do all the work for you. You will have to be the one to print that list and decide: all right, this is something that I can see myself eating and this is something that I do not see myself eating.

No one expects you to eat radishes and pumpkin seeds all day. You will have to be the one to look at both lists of foods and figure out how you will make a meal plan that works for you.

Secret 15: Make a list of all of the foods that you cannot eat on this diet.

We have tackled the most difficult part of this secret, too. We have made a list of all the acid ash foods for you, but remember, you are not banned from eating acid ash foods completely. You are still allowed 20 percent of your calories for the day from acid ash foods. Later, we will provide you with a tip that will help you easily get to this magical 20 percent number, but you have to figure out which foods from the acid ash list you would like to include in your meal plan. This will be based on your own palate and preferences.

Secret 16: If you are beginning the Alkaline Diet as a way of manipulating your pH in order to treat a specific medical problem, it may be important for you to consult your doctor before you begin this diet, informing him or her that you will be beginning a diet that involves partaking of certain foods while avoiding others. The Alkaline Diet is a safe and effective way to achieve a healthy life style and to achieve any other goals that you have, whether they are weight loss goals or involve treating a particular health concern. Because at least some of you may be embarking on this diet to treat or prevent a health problem, it is always a good idea to consult your physician first. Be aware, however, that your physician may either be unfamiliar with the Alkaline Diet or have misconceptions of the Alkaline Diet. No one is asking you to educate your physician, but it might be a good idea to explain what the Alkaline Diet means to you, or even to bring a list of the sort of foods you plan to eat. Again, this is not one of those diets where you are being asked to drink some sort of blended concoction that may cause you to pass out or have seizures or something. We are talking about coconuts, tomatoes, tofu, avocados, zucchini, grapefruit, and almonds, here, okay? These are things that are perfectly healthy and natural and which many of you are probably already eating or should be.

Secret 17: As in any diet, it is always a good idea to let significant others, family, or anyone that you live with that you are beginning a diet and therefore will be avoiding certain foods as part of your diet. This is a secret to success on any diet, but it is particularly important in the Alkaline Diet as many people that you know are most likely unfamiliar with this diet. Even if they have heard of it, they probably do not really understand it, as there are even some healthcare providers that do not.

What you want to do here is to explain to your significant others that you will be beginning a diet that focuses on eating some foods while avoiding others in order to help your body achieve homeostasis more easily and prevent certain health problems. It really should not be that difficult for most people to understand. You can explain that the foods that we eat have an effect on the pH of our blood and extracellular fluids and that the goal of your diet is to shift your pH toward the alkaline or basic end of the spectrum to prevent conditions that are associated with acidosis and improve your overall health. See? That was easy, wasn't it?

Secret 18: Most likely your kitchen contains many foods that are no-nos on your diet. An important step for you in beginning this diet will be to throughout any acidotic or acid ash foods as will derail you from your diet and exacerbate any condition that you may be attempting to treat with your diet.This is another dietary secret that is very important on the Alkaline Diet is this diet has a clear regimen of foods that should be avoided.

Over time you will get a sense of what foods are alkaline ash and which foods tend to be acid ash, but no one is expecting you to understand that just starting out. For this reason, it may be a good idea to consult the list that we provided to help you rifle through the contents of your kitchen and figure out which foods you are going to keep and which foods are ingredients you may, perhaps, choose to part with. Again, you do not have to get rid of all the acid ash foods and ingredients as you are allowed some acid ash foods in the day, but it may be easier for you to consider parting with at least some of them if you think they may derail you from success on this healthy diet.

Secret 19: If you have not already done so, get into the habit of reading labels on foods. This is not only for caloric reasons, but also to get a sense of which foods are heavily processed and contain acids that will counteract the acid ash foods you are eating. Most labels clearly identify when a food contains acids.

The labels are not lying! There are really acids, people! Although we have done the hard part for you in making detailed lists of which foods are acid ash foods and which foods are alkaline ash foods, success on this diet will, in part, be dictated by how well you understand what the diet is attempting to do and what the composition of the foods that we eat are. In other words, this diet should not be like completing an essay for school; it should be part of a new lifestyle that you are developing for yourself. Once you have started to read food labels (if you haven't started this already), you will likely be fascinated by what all goes into our foods, specifically how many acids and preservatives companies put in there.

This is a secret that most companies engaged in the food business don't want you to know. They don't want you reading labels. If you actually understood what was in the packaged food that you eat, you probably would only shop at farmer's markets or move to a remote island or something. Ignorance is bliss, as they say, but part of this diet involves educating yourself about what you are putting into your body.

Secret 20: An easy way to make sure you are getting at least 80% of your foods in a day from alkaline ash sources is by dividing all of your three meals for the day into two portions (so a total of six meals). Devote one of those six portions to an acid ash food, like a meat, fish, or non-alkaline grain. If the rest of your food portions are from alkaline acid foods then you have achieved your proper ratio.

Now, this is a fun secret because it really seems like a secret that even some of you that have engaged on the Alkaline Diet haven't tried. A question that some people will have is, how can I figure out how to get 20 percent of my calories from acid ash? And it is a good question.

The most in depth approach to answering this question would be to explain portion sizes and, in general, how big an ounce of this or that is, but the simplest way to answer this question is to use the trick that we utilized above. Twenty percent is one-fifth and in the example above we use one-sixth as a close approximation. If you divide all of your food for the day into five or six portions, you can merely set aside one of those portions as a primarily acid ash portion. So perhaps one portion will be that steak taco from your local taqueria that you have been craving all day. Again, no one is saying that you cannot consume acid ash foods ever, you just need to know what acid ash foods are and make attempts to limit them to no more than 20 percent of your calories for the day.

Secret 21: The Alkaline Diet is something that the ancients understood even if they really did not know about pH. So sit back and enjoy the well-being that comes with eating healthily and lengthening your lifespan in a natural, time-proven way.

This is the true secret to the Alkaline Diet and many other diets that dieters love. Most diets were not really invented in the last fifty or one hundred years, it's just that we understand science better now so we can apply science to principles or ideas that have been around for ages. All around the world human beings have developed a sense of what sorts of foods were better than others, even what sorts of foods can help treat this condition or that. Even with all of our modern medical and research technology we cannot always figure out how this food or natural ingredient is able to accomplish this neat thing, much less try to figure out how someone two thousand years ago would have known that. By embarking on the Alkaline Diet, you are becoming part of an old tradition that has allowed people all around the world to live long, full lives, free of many ailments that stem from the modern diet. Embarking on this diet is the beginning of a journey that will lead to the clarity of mind that comes from leaving the modern world behind an embarking on a more natural way of life.

Chapter 6: Frequently Asked Questions

What is the Alkaline Diet? The Alkaline Diet is a nutrition program that involves consuming certain foods in order to correct or prevent certain conditions associated with acidosis (low pH) of the blood or urine. The Alkaline Diet can also be used to achieve a general sense of health and wellness, for weight loss, and to achieve increased energy. The foods that one consumes on the Alkaline Diet help to shift the body away from acidosis because these foods are on the other end of the pH spectrum, they are alkaline (high pH).

Is the Alkaline Diet safe?

The Alkaline Diet is considered safe as it consists of foods that are generally regarded as healthier than other foods consumed in many diets. Many of your heavily processed foods and drinks are acid ash foods, which can easily be determined by reading food labels. Most processed or packaged foods contain acids or other compounds that are associated with making the body more acidotic. The Alkaline Diet does not involve consuming any strange or radical formulations, merely foods that can be easily obtained at a supermarket or farmer's market. As some people may be embarking on this diet for aid with a specific health condition, it is always a good idea to consult with your doctor or healthcare provider.

Is the Alkaline Diet the same as being a vegetarian or a vegan?

This is a good question. In reality, meats and fish (carnivorous foods) are all acid ash foods, so on an Alkaline Diet you would only be allowed to have about 20 percent of your food form sources like meat or fish, though you would be able to consume certain types of milk, though not other dairy products like cheese and eggs, which are considered acid ash foods. So, to answer your question, the Alkaline Ash diet can be a type of lacto-vegetarian diet, as the only animal product you would be able to consume in the alkaline ash percentage is certain types of milk, and some people choose to avoid meat, fish, and dairy altogether.

Can I drink milk on an Alkaline Diet?

Good question. Why is it a good question? Well, because there is not a consensus about this. Cow's milk is basic with a pH of about 7.33, but this is actually lower than the physiologic pH of humans of 7.4. Some nutritionists think it's okay, indeed, many of us were taught in school that milk is basic so it's a great way to counteract the activity of spicy foods! Though milk may be basic compared to many foods in the Western diet, technically, it is still lower than physiologic pH, therefore, again, you will have to decide whether you want to consume cow's milk. Goat's milk, however, is definitely part of the Alkaline Diet, as is Almond Milk.

What is the difference between acid ash and alkaline ash?

The terms "acid ash" and "alkaline ash" refer to the pH of the ash of foods after you combust them in a food combustion machine (that reduces them to ash). That's it. Acid ash foods have an acidic pH, that is pH below about 7.3, while alkaline ash foods have a basic or alkaline pH. The reason why this is important is because acid ash and alkaline ash foods have an effect on pH within the body; therefore, alkaline ash foods can be used to help correct states associated with acidosis in the body.

How does the Alkaline Diet help people with kidney stones?

The problem with kidney stones is that the blood and the urine, specifically, are acidotic, which can be easily measured with tests that measure pH, so the utility of the Alkaline Diet in this instance is in shifting your blood and urine toward a more alkaline pH, therefore preventing your kidneys from forming kidney stones. You may already know that the formation of kidney stones is associated with consumption of diets heavy in nitrogenous, acidic foods, like meat, for example. As you know, the Alkaline Diet does not include any meat and this would help you with kidney stones.

Does the Alkaline diet involve eating organic food?

There is not a clear cut relationship between the Alkaline Diet and whether a food is organic or not, as both alkaline ash foods and acid ash foods can be organic. Indeed, any alkaline ash foods may not be organic, so if consuming organic foods is important to you then you need to carefully read food labels (or shop at farmer's markets where they sell organic food).

Can the Alkaline Diet be incorporated with other diets?

We delve into this issue more deeply in a latter question, but it is definitely possible to incorporate the Alkaline Diet with other diets. This is easily accomplished as the Alkaline Diet focuses on what you are eating, not on how much or when. As you may already know, most diets fall under the Total Caloric Restriction category, meaning that they involve eating fewer calories as a mainstay of the diet. Other diets manipulate timing of when food is consumed (Intermittent Fasting) or play around with the ratio of one nutrient versus another (Ketogenic Diet). As this diet, again, is more about eating foods that are alkaline, it is not difficult to incorporate with other diets, you would just have to make sure that you are consuming foods that are in the Alkaline category.

Do I need to measure my pH while on the Alkaline Diet?

In this eBook we went into great detail explaining what pH was and why pH is an important part of the Alkaline Diet. As a quick review, the pH is essentially what tells us if our blood or urine is acidic, basic (alkaline) or neutral. For some people, their goal on this diet is to treat or prevent conditions associated with acidosis of the blood or urine. An Alkaline diet will shift the blood and urine away from acidosis by natural means through the consumption of alkaline ash foods. Some people may choose to measure the pH of their urine on this diet, especially if their concern is kidney stones, and there are several ways that one may measure the pH of the urine. In reality, it is not essential to measure pH of the blood or urine while on this diet.

Should I consult with a physician before I begin the Alkaline Diet?

Any person considering beginning a diet should consult their physician. This is particularly true in the case of the Alkaline Diet as many of you may be embarking on this diet with a specific goal of treating a health condition. The Alkaline Diet is healthy and the foods that are part of this diet are natural and organic, but when in doubt always ask your physician or health provider for guidance.

I occasionally go on fasts. Can I fast while on the Alkaline Diet?

Fasting is perfectly healthy and natural. Indeed, human beings have been fasting for many thousands of years, for both practical reasons and for religious or spiritual reasons. In fact, periods of fasting punctuated by shorter periods of eating is the normal way that our human ancestors would have eaten and lived in the earlier days of human history. They did not have fast food and soda, they did not have refrigerators, freezers, and processed foods to keep in the cupboards. They would not even have had cupboards. If they were hungry, these early humans would have to hunt and fish to satiate that hungry. Therefore, they would have had prolonged periods were they were not eating. It is the opinion of this book that fasts as perfectly healthy and can easily be incorporated into an Alkaline Diet. Naturally, any person with an underlying health problems that affect the absorption or metabolism of food, like diabetes mellitus, should consult a doctor before beginning any diet.

How will I know if my Alkaline Diet is working?

We talk about this later in some of the other questions, but the way that you will know if your diet is working will be a function of what your goals are on the diet. Many of you will begin this diet because you just want to feel healthier and you have heard that the Alkaline Diet is a fantastic way to steer your body in a healthier direction. Others of you will embark on the Alkaline Diet because you have a specific health issue and you would like to utilize this diet as part of the management of your health condition. If your goal is general health and wellness, you would measure your success on this diet by things like increased energy, less depression and anxiety, better skin tone resulting from less processed, acidic foods, and the like. If you are engaging in this diet for a specific health reason, then you would have to continue to utilize whatever means you use to keep track of your condition.

Can I expect weight loss while on the Alkaline Diet?
Many people on the Alkaline Diet experience weight loss, and this occurs for a number of reasons. One of the main reasons is that the Alkaline Diet steers you away from processed foods or other foods that screw with your metabolism (like heavy starches). Because of this, your body has to expend fewer calories to digest food, is less likely to store excess calories as fat (because you are not eating the acid ash foods that are associated with fat storage) and reaches homeostasis a little easier than it might otherwise.

I have an active fitness regimen. Will the Alkaline Diet interfere with my ability achieve my fitness goals?
This is a common question for people starting any diet and it is a very important question to act. In general, the issue that people engaged actively in fitness will have on the Alkaline Diet is making the food requirements of this diet work for them in terms of their own macronutrient needs. Many of you active in the fitness world will have specific goals in terms of daily macronutrient consumption (fats, carbohydrates, and proteins) so you may have to make significant adjustments to your diet as many of the foods that you are used to eating will be acid ash foods. It is completely possible to meet your macronutrient goals while on an Alkaline Diet, though those of you with extremely high protein demands may have to make

an adjustment. You can maintain a healthy protein intake while on the Alkaline Diet, but as this diet avoids the acid ash foods of most meats and dairy, then you would have to find other sources for your protein and possibly lower you protein quota a bit.

Is it difficult to stick to an Alkaline Diet?

It is not easy sticking to any diet. If it was, everyone would partake of diets and we all would achieve are dietary goals. In reality, many people who embark on diets fail and this is often a function of having unrealistic expectations on the diet or not being disciplined enough to stick to the diet. Fortunately for many people, the Alkaline Diet includes many foods that people enjoy eating and the problem is not so much sticking to the diet, so to speak, but getting used to not eating foods that one may be used to eating, like sour or bitter fruits, meats, grains, and the like. In reality, it is no more difficult to stick to the diet than it is to stick to any other diet; indeed, it may be a bit easier as you are not restricting your caloric intake on this diet (unless you want to) as you would be on many other diets, like a Low Fat diet, or any other diet that involves Total Caloric Restriction.

What are the advantages of the Alkaline Diet compared to other diets?

This is not a simple question as ever dieter has their own individual reasons that determine why they choose to go on a diet in the first place, and why they might choose one particular diet over another. Many individuals that choose to go on a "diet" do so because their goal is weight loss or fat loss. In reality, a "diet" is nothing more than a specific eating regimen, therefore the goal of a diet does not have to be weight loss or fat loss. If the goal of your diet is, in fact, weight loss the Alkaline Diet can help you achieve weight loss as the foods that are the staples of this diet are generally associated with less storage of excess calories in the form of fat, as well as improved metabolism and insulin resistance. These latter benefits are achieved on the Alkaline Diet as this diet does not include the grains and heavily processed foods that tend to steer us toward weight gain. Many other diets, however, can help you achieve your goal if your goal is weight loss. Diets that have been shown to be effective at weight loss include Intermittent Fasting, the Ketogenic Diet (of which Atkins is a type), and perhaps the most common diet, Total Caloric Restriction. Total Caloric Restriction is nothing more than the general term for a diet that is based around reducing your overall caloric intake in order to put you in a caloric deficit and encourage your body to burn fat for energy.

Though the Alkaline Diet can trigger weight loss, its advantages vis a vis other diets have more to do with its health benefits. The Alkaline Diet has been shown to prevent and also treat kidney stones, muscle wasting, osteoporosis, and various other diets associated with acidosis of the blood or urine. The Alkaline Diet helps the body maintain homeostasis, which is often difficult in the modern Western diet of processed foods and sodas that are acid ash foods that shift the blood toward acidosis and encourage harmful conditions like osteoporosis. Therefore, it is difficult to compare the Alkaline Diet to other diets as the goals of dieters in this particular diet are generally different from those in other diets.

What do I need to do to be successful on my Alkaline Diet?

A major component of being successful on a diet, including this one, is having a clear idea of your goals on this diet, as well as an idea of how you plan to accomplish those goals. As your plan as far as accomplishing your goals essentially involves following this diet to a "T", this e-book will do some of the work for you. If you plan to follow the Alkaline Diet closely, all you really need to do is eat the foods that fall under the alkaline ash category and avoid the acid ash foods. Another component of being successful on a diet is having a sense of how you are going to measure your goals. For example, if your goal on your diet is weight loss then naturally you need to make sure that you weight yourself on the first day of your diet and, say, once a week thereafter. As this is an Alkaline Diet that we are talking about, many of you will have goals that involve a health condition perhaps or the prevention of a health condition. Therefore it might be more obvious to you if you are meeting your goals on this diet as the symptoms associated with your condition would diminish or disappear completely. And finally, people often feel healthier and more energetic on an Alkaline Diet as their body does not have to expend so much energy digesting food or keeping the body in homeostasis, so you should notice yourself feeling a little better on this diet. This is an indication of success, as well.

What is the approach of the medical community to the Alkaline Diet?

Good question. There is some controversy surrounding the Alkaline Diet in the medical community, primarily as there has been an assertion that some of the claims of the Alkaline Diet have not been verified. Although not every claim made by advocates of this diet has been backed by medical research, in reality, there is actually overlap between much of the ideas that are part of the Alkaline Diet and suggestions made by doctors themselves. For example, doctors will normally advise people suffering from kidney stones to avoid certain foods and dietary practices, like consuming meals heavy with meats, and this is actually an important aspect of the Alkaline Diet as meats are considered acid ash foods. The long and short of it, there is not agreement between the medical and dietetic communities as far as this diet is concerned, although there is significant overlap between the suggestions made by both camps.

Conclusion

Thank you for purchasing *Alkaline Diet for Beginners,* In this book, we gave you an in-depth look at the ins and outs of the Alkaline Diet, explaining all of the science behind pH and why an understanding of pH is important to this diet. Although you do not have to measure your pH in order to begin or be successful on the Alkaline Diet, we do find that someone who understand why their diet works or why they should consume some foods rather than others is more likely to achieve success on this diet. As an important component to understanding this diet was understanding some of the health problems that the Alkaline Diet can treat, we took you on a whirlwind tour of several health problems that are influenced by pH and explained how certain foods can help to remedy these problems. Of course, being successful on any diet requires understanding exactly what you can eat and what you can't, so we gave you a clear and concise breakdown of the alkaline ash foods and the acid ash foods to enable you to easily achieve the proper ratio on your Alkaline Diet.

We understand that the Alkaline Ash Diet will be unfamiliar to many people, so we made sure not to leave you hanging with just the facts. We distilled the facts contained in this book to 21 secrets that you can use to achieve weight loss, increased energy, or whatever other goals you are seeking on your Alkaline Diet. Finally, because pretty much everyone will have a host of questions before they embark on their diet, we provided you with a list of the most common questions dieters generally have about the Alkaline Diet.

Again, we thank you for purchasing this book. We wish you all the success in the world in approaching this diet like Superman approaches another day in Metropolis. We know that you will find all the success that you are hoping for, and we encourage you to refer back to this book whenever you find yourself with questions about your new diet.

CPSIA information can be obtained
at www.ICGtesting.com
Printed in the USA
BVHW072301291020
592123BV00014B/2067